The Best Mediterranean Cookbook for Pros

Easy Healthy Dinner Recipes -

Eleanor Bidell

Sommario

Introduction

Thinking of the principle of diet plan in current times we promptly think of drastic diets such as fasting or ketogenic diet plan, however our publication will certainly offer much more, our publication is based upon fat burning guaranteed with our Mediterranean diet plan, which is not based upon a radical reduction of calories but at the same time you do not need to give up the swimwear examination.

A false belief of modern-day diet regimens is the impossibility of eating snak or desserts but thanks to this diet you will certainly see that it is absolutely not so, enjoy delighting in these dishes for you as well as your household without quiting weight loss and far better physical stamina.

If you are hesitant about this fantastic diet regimen you simply have to try it and evaluate your results in a short time, believe me you will certainly be pleased.

Always keep in mind that the most effective way to lose weight is to evaluate your circumstance with the help of an expert.

Appreciate.

Mediterranean Diet Lunch Recipes

Broccoli and Carrots Soup

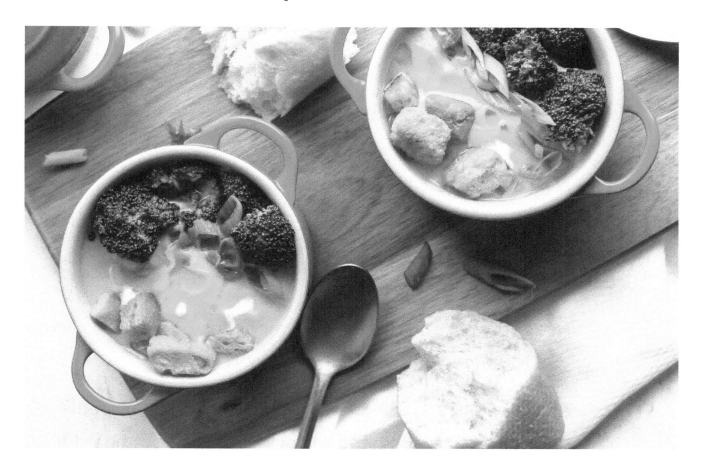

Prep time: 10 minutes I **Cooking time:** 25 minutes I **Servings:** 4

Ingredients:

- 2 carrots, peeled and grated

- 1 pound broccoli florets

- 1 yellow onion, chopped

- 2 garlic cloves, minced

- 1 tablespoon olive oil

- 1 teaspoon chili powder

- 4 cups veggie stock

- 1 teaspoon ginger, grated

- Juice of 1 lime

- A pinch of salt and black pepper

- 1 tablespoon parsley, chopped

Directions:

1. Heat up a pot with the oil over medium heat, add the onion and the garlic and sauté for 5 minutes.

2. Add the carrots, the broccoli and the other ingredients, toss, bring to a simmer and cook over medium heat for 20 minutes more.

3. Divide the soup into bowls and serve.

Nutrition facts per serving: calories 108, fat 6.1, fiber 4.6, carbs 16.4, protein 4

Tomato Soup

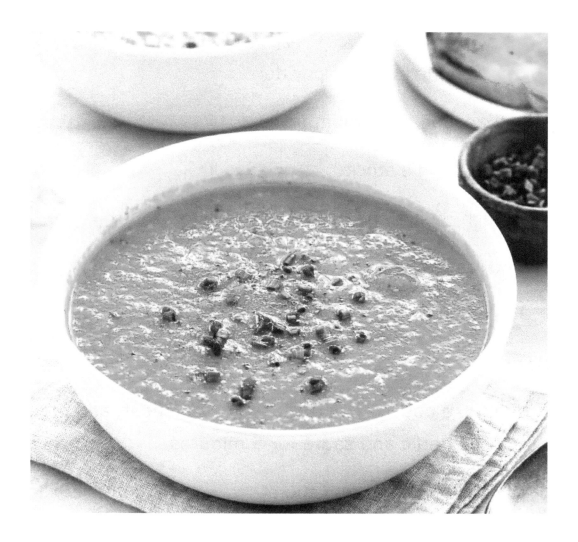

Prep time: 5 minutes I **Cooking time:** 25 minutes I **Servings:** 4

Ingredients:

- 1 yellow onion, chopped

- 2 tablespoons olive oil

- 2 garlic cloves, minced

- 1 pound tomatoes, cubed

- 2 teaspoons turmeric powder

- ¼ teaspoon cardamom powder

- 5 cups veggie stock

- A pinch of salt and black pepper

- 6 ounces baby spinach

- 2 teaspoons lime juice

Directions:

1. Heat up a pot with the oil over medium heat, add the onion and the garlic and sauté for 5 minutes.

2. Add the tomatoes and the other ingredients, toss, simmer over medium heat for 20 minutes more, ladle into bowls and serve.

Nutrition facts per serving: calories 123, fat 10.1, fiber 3.3, carbs 13.3, protein 2.8

Tuna Bowls

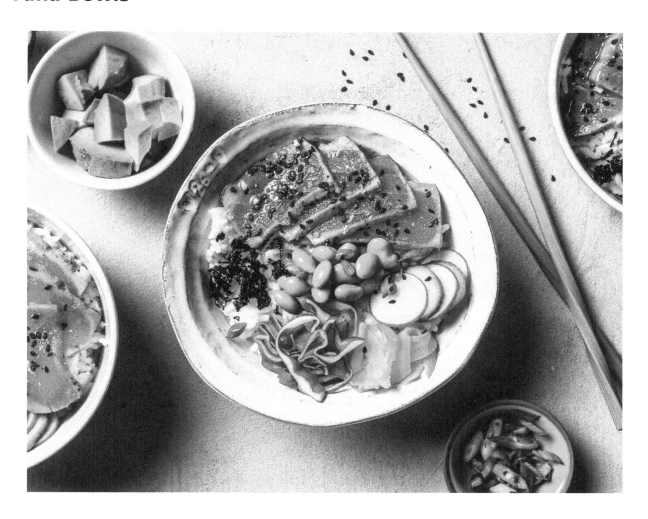

Prep time: 10 minutes I **Cooking time:** 25 minutes I **Servings:** 4

Ingredients:

- 2 cups quinoa, cooked

- ½ cup tomato puree

- 3 ounces smoked tuna, boneless and flaked

- 1 yellow onion, chopped

- 1 tablespoon olive oil

- 1 teaspoon sweet paprika

- 2 teaspoons turmeric powder

- A pinch of salt and black pepper

- 1 tablespoon chives, chopped

Directions:

1. Heat up a pan with the oil over medium heat, add the onion and sauté for 5 minutes.

2. Add the quinoa, the tuna and the remaining ingredients, toss, cook for 20 minutes more, divide into bowls and serve.

Nutrition facts per serving: calories 411, fat 10.7, fiber 7.6, carbs 61, protein 18.7

Trout and Asparagus

Prep time: 5 minutes I **Cooking time:** 20 minutes I **Servings:** 4

Ingredients:

- 4 trout fillets, boneless

- 1 yellow onion, chopped

- 2 tablespoons olive oil

- 1 bunch asparagus, halved and trimmed

- 3 tablespoons balsamic vinegar

- 1 tablespoon mustard

- 1 garlic clove, minced

- 1 tablespoon chives, chopped

- A pinch of salt and black pepper

Directions:

1. Heat up a pan with the oil over medium-high heat, add the onion and the asparagus and sauté for 3 minutes.

2. Add the fish and sear it for 2 minutes on each side.

3. Add the remaining ingredients, bake everything in the oven at 360 for 13 minutes more, divide everything between plates and serve for lunch.

Nutrition facts per serving: calories 266, fat 11, fiber 6, carbs 14.2, protein 9

Shrimp Bowls

Prep time: 10 minutes I **Cooking time:** 20 minutes I **Servings:** 4

Ingredients:

- 1 yellow onion, chopped

- 1 tablespoon olive oil

- 1 pound shrimp, peeled and deveined

- 1 cup mushrooms, sliced

- ½ cup chicken stock

- A pinch of salt and black pepper

- 1 teaspoon turmeric powder

- 1 tablespoon oregano, chopped

Directions:

1. Heat up a pan with the oil over medium heat, add the onion and the mushrooms, stir and sauté for 10 minutes.

2. Add the shrimp and the other ingredients, toss, cook everything for 10 minutes more, divide into bowls and serve.

Nutrition facts per serving: calories 261, fat 7, fiber 8, carbs 8.6, protein 7.1

Shrimp with Parsley and Quinoa

Prep time: 5 minutes I **Cooking time:** 10 minutes I **Servings:** 4

Ingredients:

- 2 garlic cloves, peeled

- 1 yellow onion, chopped

- 1 pound shrimp, peeled and deveined

- 1 tablespoon olive oil

- 1 cup cherry tomatoes, cut into quarters

- 2 cups quinoa, cooked

- 1 tablespoon parsley, chopped

- 1 teaspoon turmeric powder

- A pinch of salt and black pepper

- A pinch of cayenne pepper

Directions:

1. Heat up a pan with the oil over medium-high heat, add the onion and the garlic and sauté for 2 minutes.

2. Add the tomatoes and sauté for 3 minutes more.

3. Add the shrimp, the quinoa and the rest of the ingredients, toss, cook for 5 minutes more, divide into bowls and serve.

Nutrition facts per serving: calories 261, fat 4, fiber 7, carbs 15, protein 7

Garlic Chicken Mix

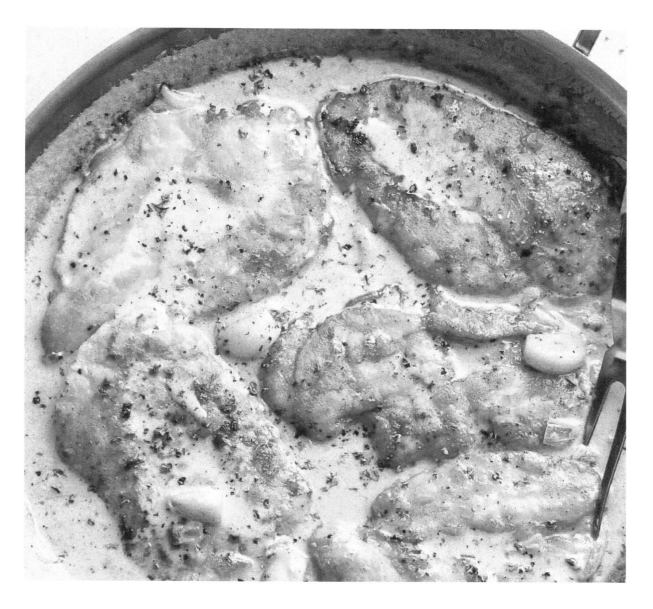

Prep time: 10 minutes I **Cooking time:** 40 minutes I **Servings:** 4

Ingredients:

- 2 sweet potatoes, peeled and cut into wedges

- 1 pound chicken breast, skinless, boneless and sliced

- 2 tablespoons olive oil

- 2 scallions, chopped

- A pinch of salt and black pepper

- 2 garlic cloves, minced

- Juice of 1 lime

- ½ cup chicken stock

Directions:

1. In a roasting pan, combine the chicken with the sweet potatoes, the oil and the other ingredients, toss gently and cook at 360 degrees F for 40 minutes.

2. Divide the mix between plates and serve.

Nutrition facts per serving: calories 222, fat 6, fiber 7, carbs 15, protein 7

Spiced Chicken Soup

Prep time: 10 minutes I **Cooking time:** 1 hour I **Servings:** 8

Ingredients:

- 1 yellow onion, chopped
- 1 pound chicken breast, skinless, boneless and cubed
- 1 tablespoon olive oil
- 2 carrots, sliced
- 3 garlic cloves, minced
- A pinch of salt and black pepper
- 6 cups veggie stock
- 2 teaspoons turmeric powder
- Juice of 1 lime
- Zest of 1 lime, grated
- 1 tablespoon cilantro, chopped

Directions:

1. Heat up a pot with the oil over medium heat, add the onion, carrots and the garlic and sauté for 5 minutes.

2. Add the meat and brown it for 5 minutes more.

3. Add the stock and the other ingredients except the cilantro, toss, bring to a simmer and cook over medium heat for 50 minutes.

4. Divide the soup into bowls, sprinkle the cilantro on top and serve.

Nutrition facts per serving: calories 271, fat 8, fiber 11, carbs 16, protein 8

Spinach and Tomato Soup

Prep time: 10 minutes I **Cooking time:** 20 minutes I **Servings:** 4

Ingredients:

- 1 pound spinach leaves

- 1 yellow onion, chopped

- 1 tablespoon olive oil

- 4 cups chicken stock

- 4 cherry tomatoes, halved

- 1 red bell pepper, chopped

- 1 tablespoon parsley, chopped

Directions:

1. Heat up a pot with the oil over medium-high heat, add the onion and the bell pepper and sauté for 5 minutes.

2. Add the spinach and the other ingredients, toss, bring to a simmer and cook over medium heat for 15 minutes.

3. Ladle the soup into bowls and serve for lunch.

Nutrition facts per serving: calories 148, fat 2, fiber 6, carbs 8, protein 5

Turkey Meatballs

Prep time: 10 minutes I **Cooking time:** 10 minutes I **Servings:** 4

Ingredients:

- 1 pound turkey meat, ground

- 1 yellow onion, chopped

- 1 egg, whisked

- 1 tablespoon cilantro, chopped

- 2 tablespoons olive oil

- 1 red chili pepper, minced

- 2 teaspoons lime juice

- Zest of 1 lime, grated

- A pinch of salt and black pepper

- 1 teaspoon turmeric powder

Directions:

1. In a bowl, combine the turkey meat with the onion and the other ingredients except the oil, stir and shape medium meatballs out of this mix.

2. Heat up a pan with the oil over medium-high heat, add the meatballs, cook them for 5 minutes on each side, divide between plates and serve for lunch.

Nutrition facts per serving: calories 200, fat 12, fiber 5, carbs 12, protein 7

Cauliflower and Tomato Soup

Prep time: 10 minutes I **Cooking time:** 35 minutes I **Servings:** 4

Ingredients:

- 1 yellow onion, chopped

- 1 carrot, chopped

- ½ cup celery, chopped

- 1 tablespoon olive oil

- 1 pound cauliflower florets

- A pinch of salt and black pepper

- 1 red bell pepper, chopped

- 5 cups vegetable stock

- 15 ounces tomatoes, chopped

- 1 tablespoon cilantro, chopped

Directions:

1. Heat up a pot with the oil over medium-high heat, add the onion, celery, carrot and the bell pepper and sauté for 10 minutes.

2. Add the cauliflower and the other ingredients, toss, bring to a simmer and cook over medium heat for 25 minutes more.

3. Ladle the soup into bowls and serve.

Nutrition facts per serving: calories 210, fat 1, fiber 5, carbs 14, protein 6

Lemon Cod Mix

Prep time: 10 minutes I **Cooking time:** 25 minutes I **Servings:** 4

Ingredients:

- 4 cod fillets, skinless

- 2 garlic cloves, minced

- 2 shallots, chopped

- Salt and black pepper to the taste

- 2 tablespoons olive oil

- 2 tablespoons tarragon, chopped

- ½ cup black olives, pitted and halved

- Juice of 1 lemon

- ¼ cup chicken stock

- 1 tablespoon chives, chopped

Directions:

1. Heat up a pan with the oil over medium-high heat, add the shallots and the garlic and sauté for 5 minutes.

2. Add the fish and sear it for 2 minutes on each side.

3. Add the remaining ingredients, put the pan in the oven and cook at 360 degrees F for 15 minutes.

4. Divide the mix between plates and serve for lunch.

Nutrition facts per serving: calories 173, fat 3, fiber 4, carbs 9, protein 12

Kale and Lemon Soup

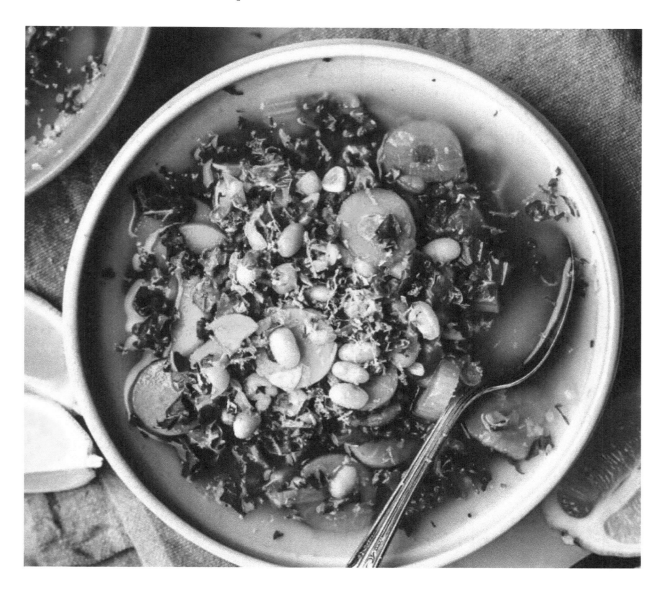

Prep time: 10 minutes I **Cooking time:** 15 minutes I **Servings:**
4

Ingredients:

- 1 pound kale, chopped

- Salt and black pepper to the taste

- 5 cups vegetable stock

- 2 carrots, sliced

- 1 yellow onion, chopped

- 1 tablespoon olive oil

- 1 tablespoon parsley, chopped

- 1 tablespoon lemon juice

Directions:

1. Heat up a pot with the oil over medium heat, add the carrots and the onion, stir and sauté for 5 minutes.

2. Add the kale and the other ingredients, toss, bring to a simmer and cook over medium heat for 10 minutes more.

3. Ladle the soup into bowls and serve.

Nutrition facts per serving: calories 210, fat 7, fiber 2, carbs 10, protein 8

Balsamic Salmon Mix

Prep time: 10 minutes I **Cooking time:** 20 minutes I **Servings:** 4

Ingredients:

- 4 salmon fillets, boneless
- 1 tablespoon olive oil
- 2 fennel bulbs, shredded
- 1 tablespoon balsamic vinegar
- 1 tablespoon lime juice
- ½ teaspoon cumin, ground
- ½ teaspoon oregano, dried
- 1 tablespoon chives, chopped
- Salt and black pepper to the taste

Directions:

1. Heat up a pan with the oil over medium heat, add the fennel, stir and sauté for 5 minutes.

2. Add the fish and sear it for 2 minutes on each side.

3. Add the remaining ingredients, cook everything for 10 minutes more, divide between plates and serve.

Nutrition facts per serving: calories 200, fat 2, fiber 4, carbs 10, protein 8

Turmeric Carrot Soup

Prep time: 10 minutes I **Cooking time:** 25 minutes I **Servings:** 4

Ingredients:

- 1 pound carrots, peeled and sliced
- 2 tablespoons olive oil
- 1 yellow onion, chopped
- 1 teaspoon rosemary, dried
- 1 teaspoon cumin, ground
- 2 garlic cloves, minced
- A pinch of salt and black pepper
- 5 cups vegetable stock
- ½ teaspoon turmeric powder
- 1 cup coconut milk
- 1 tablespoon chives, chopped

Directions:

1. Heat up a pot with the oil over medium heat, add the onion and the garlic and sauté for 5 minutes.

2. Add the carrots, the stock and the other ingredients except the chives, stir, bring to a simmer and cook over medium heat for 20 minutes more.

3. Divide the soup into bowls, sprinkle the chives on top and serve for lunch.

Nutrition facts per serving: calories 210, fat 8, fiber 6, carbs 10, protein 7

Coconut Leeks Soup

Prep time: 10 minutes I **Cooking time:** 20 minutes I **Servings:** 4

Ingredients:

- 4 leeks, sliced

- 1 yellow onion, chopped

- 1 tablespoon avocado oil

- A pinch of salt and black pepper

- 2 garlic cloves, minced

- 4 cups vegetable soup

- ½ cup coconut milk

- ½ teaspoon nutmeg, ground

- ¼ teaspoon red pepper, crushed

- ½ teaspoon rosemary, dried

- 1 tablespoon parsley, chopped

Directions:

1. Heat up a pot with the oil over medium-high heat, add the onion and the garlic and sauté for 2 minutes.

2. Add the leeks, stir and sauté for 3 minutes more.

3. Add the stock and the rest of the ingredients except the parsley, bring to a simmer and cook over medium heat for 15 minutes more.

4. Blend the soup with an immersion blender, divide the soup into bowls, sprinkle the parsley on top and serve.

Nutrition facts per serving: calories 268, fat 11.8, fiber 4.5, carbs 37.4, protein 6.1

Paprika Turkey Mix

Prep time: 10 minutes I **Cooking time:** 40 minutes I **Servings:** 4

Ingredients:

- 1 yellow onion, sliced

- 1 pound turkey breast, skinless, boneless and roughly cubed

- 2 tablespoons olive oil

- Salt and black pepper to the taste

- 1 cup artichoke hearts, halved

- ½ teaspoon nutmeg, ground

- ½ teaspoon sweet paprika

- 1 teaspoon cumin, ground

- 1 tablespoon cilantro, chopped

Directions:

1. In a roasting pan, combine the turkey with the onion, artichokes and the other ingredients, toss and at 350 degrees F for 40 minutes.

2. Divide everything between plates and serve.

Nutrition facts per serving: calories 345, fat 12, fiber 3, carbs 12, protein 14

Salmon and Spinach Salad

Prep time: 10 minutes I **Cooking time:** 0 minutes I **Servings:** 4

Ingredients:

- 2 cups smoked salmon, skinless, boneless and cut into strips
- 1 yellow onion, chopped
- 1 avocado, peeled, pitted and cubed
- 1 cup cherry tomatoes, halved
- 1 tablespoon olive oil
- 2 cups baby spinach
- A pinch of salt and cayenne pepper
- 1 tablespoon balsamic vinegar

Directions:

1. In a salad bowl, mix the salmon with the onion, the avocado and the other ingredients, toss, divide between plates and serve for lunch.

Nutrition facts per serving: calories 260, fat 2, fiber 8, carbs 17, protein 11

Turmeric Shrimp

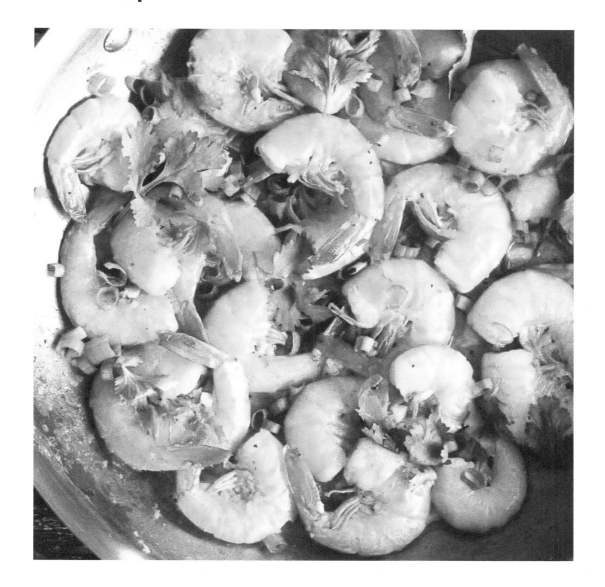

Prep time: 10 minutes I **Cooking time:** 17 minutes I **Servings:** 4

Ingredients:

- 1 pound shrimp, peeled and deveined

- 1 tablespoon lemon juice

- 2 zucchinis, sliced

- 1 yellow onion, roughly chopped

- 1 tablespoon olive oil

- 1 teaspoon turmeric powder

- A pinch of salt and black pepper

- 1 tablespoons capers, drained

- 2 tablespoons pine nuts

Directions:

1. Heat up a pan with the oil over medium-high heat, add the onion and the zucchini, stir and sauté for 5 minutes.

2. Add the shrimp and the other ingredients, toss, cook everything for 12 minutes more, divide into bowls and serve for lunch.

Nutrition facts per serving: calories 162, fat 3, fiber 4, carbs 12, protein 7

Broccoli Stew

Prep time: 10 minutes I **Cooking time:** 25 minutes I **Servings:** 4

Ingredients:

- 1 tablespoon olive oil

- 1 pound broccoli florets

- ½ teaspoon coriander, ground

- 1 yellow onion, chopped

- 2 leeks, sliced

- 4 garlic cloves, minced

- ½ teaspoon turmeric powder

- A pinch of cayenne pepper

- 1 cup tomato paste

- A pinch of salt and black pepper

- 1 tablespoon lemon juice

- 1 tablespoon cilantro, chopped

Directions:

1. Heat up a pot with the oil over medium heat, add the onion, garlic, leeks and the turmeric and sauté for 5 minutes.

2. Add the broccoli and the other ingredients, toss, bring to a simmer and cook over medium heat for 25 minutes more.

3. Divide into bowls and serve for lunch.

Nutrition facts per serving: calories 113, fat 4.1, fiber 4.5, carbs 17.7, protein 4.4

Salmon with Garlic Green Beans

Prep time: 10 minutes I **Cooking time:** 26 minutes I **Servings:** 4

Ingredients:

- 2 tablespoons olive oil

- 1 yellow onion, chopped

- 4 salmon fillets, boneless

- 1 cup green beans, trimmed and halved

- 2 garlic cloves, minced

- ½ cup chicken stock

- 1 teaspoon chili powder

- 1 teaspoon sweet paprika

- A pinch of salt and black pepper

- 1 tablespoon cilantro, chopped

Directions:

1. Heat up a pan with the oil over medium heat, add onion, stir and sauté for 2 minutes.

2. Add the fish and sear it for 2 minutes on each side.

3. Add the rest of the ingredients, toss gently and bake everything at 360 degrees F for 20 minutes.

4. Divide everything between plates and serve for lunch.

Nutrition facts per serving: calories 322, fat 18.3, fiber 2, carbs 5.8, protein 35.7

Coconut Chicken Stew

Prep time: 10 minutes I **Cooking time:** 45 minutes I **Servings:** 4

Ingredients:

- 1 tablespoon olive oil

- 1 pound chicken thighs, skinless, boneless and cubed

- 2 garlic cloves, minced

- 1 small yellow onion, chopped

- 1 green bell pepper, chopped

- 1 red bell pepper, chopped

- ½ teaspoon cumin, ground

- ½ teaspoon sweet paprika

- 2 cups chicken stock

- A pinch of salt and black pepper

- 1 tablespoon lemon juice

- 1 cup coconut milk

- 1 tablespoon cilantro, chopped

Directions:

1. Heat up a pot with the oil over medium heat, add the onion, garlic and the meat and brown for 10 minutes stirring often.

2. Add the rest of the ingredients except the coconut milk and the cilantro, stir, bring to a simmer and cook over medium for 30 minutes more.

3. Add the coconut milk and the cilantro, stir, simmer the stew for 5 minutes more, divide into bowls and serve for lunch.

Nutrition facts per serving: calories 419, fat 26.8, fiber 2.7, carbs 10.7, protein 35.5

Lemon Turkey Stew

Prep time: 10 minutes I **Cooking time:** 45 minutes I **Servings:**
6

Ingredients:

- 1 pound turkey breast, skinless, boneless and cubed

- 1 yellow onion, chopped

- 2 tablespoons olive oil

- ½ teaspoon mustard seeds

- 1 teaspoon ginger, grated

- 2 garlic cloves, minced

- 1 green chili pepper, chopped

- 1 teaspoon sweet paprika

- 1 teaspoon coriander, ground

- ½ teaspoon cardamom, ground

- ½ teaspoon turmeric powder

- A pinch of salt and black pepper

- 1 teaspoon lemon juice

- 1 cup chicken stock

- 1 tablespoon parsley, chopped

Directions:

1. Heat up a pot with the oil over medium-high heat, add the onion, the meat, mustard seeds, ginger, garlic, paprika, coriander, cardamom and the turmeric, stir and brown for 10 minutes.

2. Add all the other ingredients, toss, simmer over medium heat for 35 minutes more, divide into bowls and serve.

Nutrition facts per serving: calories 202, fat 9.4, fiber 1.7, carbs 9.3, protein 20.3

Beef Pan

Prep time: 5 minutes I **Cooking time:** 20 minutes I **Servings:** 4

Ingredients:

- 1 pound beef, ground

- ½ cup yellow onion, chopped

- 1 tablespoon olive oil

- 1 cup zucchini, cubed

- 2 garlic cloves, minced

- 14 ounces tomatoes, chopped

- 1 teaspoon Italian seasoning

- ¼ cup parmesan, shredded

- 1 tablespoon chives, chopped

- 1 tablespoon cilantro, chopped

Directions:

1. Heat up a pan with the oil over medium heat, add the garlic, onion and the beef and brown for 5 minutes.

2. Add the rest of the ingredients, toss, cook for 15 minutes more, divide into bowls and serve for lunch.

Nutrition facts per serving: calories 276, fat 11.3, fiber 1.9, carbs 6.8, protein 36

Thyme Beef

Prep time: 10 minutes I **Cooking time:** 25 minutes I **Servings:** 4

Ingredients:

- ½ pound beef, ground

- 3 tablespoons olive oil

- 1 and ¾ pounds red potatoes, peeled and roughly cubed

- 1 yellow onion, chopped

- 2 teaspoons thyme, dried

- 1 cup tomatoes, chopped

- A pinch of black pepper

Directions:

1. Heat up a pan with the oil over medium-high heat, add the onion and the beef, stir and brown for 5 minutes.

2. Add the potatoes and the rest of the ingredients, toss, bring to a simmer, cook for 20 minutes more, divide into bowls and serve for lunch.

Nutrition facts per serving: calories 216, fat 14.5, fiber 5.2, carbs 40.7, protein 22.2

Pork Soup

Prep time: 10 minutes I **Cooking time:** 25 minutes I **Servings:** 4

Ingredients:

- 1 tablespoon olive oil

- 1 red onion, chopped

- 1 pound pork stew meat, cubed

- 1 quart beef stock

- 1 pound carrots, sliced

- 1 cup tomato puree

- 1 tablespoon cilantro, chopped

Directions:

1. Heat up a pot with the oil over medium-high heat, add the onion and the meat and brown for 5 minutes.

2. Add the rest of the ingredients except the cilantro, bring to a simmer, reduce heat to medium, and boil the soup for 20 minutes.

3. Ladle into bowls and serve for lunch with the cilantro sprinkled on top.

Nutrition facts per serving: calories 354, fat 14.6, fiber 4.6, carbs 19.3, protein 36

Shrimp and Corn Salad

Prep time: 5 minutes I **Cooking time:** 7 minutes I **Servings:** 4

Ingredients:

- 1 cup corn

- 1 endive, shredded

- 1 cup baby spinach

- 1 pound shrimp, peeled and deveined

- 2 garlic cloves, minced

- 1 tablespoon lime juice

- 2 cups strawberries, halved

- 2 tablespoons olive oil

- 2 tablespoons balsamic vinegar

- 1 tablespoon cilantro, chopped

Directions:

1. Heat up a pan with the oil over medium-high heat, add the garlic and brown for 1 minute. Add the shrimp and lime juice, toss and cook for 3 minutes on each side.

2. In a salad bowl, combine the shrimp with the corn, endive and the other ingredients, toss and serve for lunch.

Nutrition facts per serving: calories 260, fat 9.7, fiber 2.9, carbs 16.5, protein 28

Raspberry Shrimp Salad

Prep time: 5 minutes I **Cooking time:** 10 minutes I **Servings:** 4

Ingredients:

- 1 pound green beans, trimmed and halved

- 2 tablespoons olive oil

- 2 pounds shrimp, peeled and deveined

- 1 tablespoon lemon juice

- 2 cups cherry tomatoes, halved

- ¼ cup raspberry vinegar

- A pinch of black pepper

Directions:

1. Heat up a pan with the oil over medium-high heat, add the shrimp, toss and cook for 2 minutes.

2. Add the green beans and the other ingredients, toss, cook for 8 minutes more, divide into bowls and serve for lunch.

Nutrition facts per serving: calories 385, fat 11.2, fiber 5, carbs 15.3, protein 54.5

Tacos

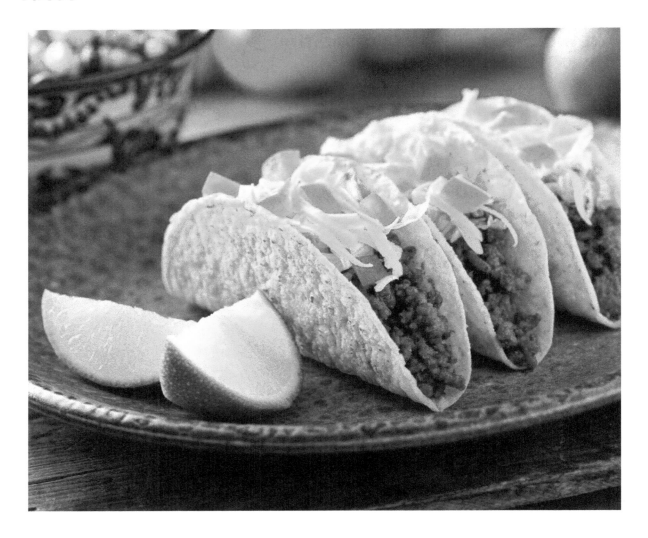

Prep time: 10 minutes I **Cooking time:** 10 minutes I **Servings:** 2

Ingredients:

- 4 whole wheat taco shells

- 1 tablespoon light mayonnaise

- 1 tablespoon salsa

- 1 tablespoon mozzarella, shredded

- 1 tablespoon olive oil

- 1 red onion, chopped

- 1 tablespoon cilantro, chopped

- 2 cod fillets, boneless, skinless and cubed

- 1 tablespoon tomato puree

Directions:

1. Heat up a pan with the oil over medium heat, add the onion, stir and cook for 2 minutes.

2. Add the fish and tomato puree, toss gently and cook for 5 minutes more.

3. Spoon this into the taco shells, also divide the mayo, salsa and the cheese and serve for lunch.

Nutrition facts per serving: calories 466, fat 14.5, fiber 8, carbs 56.6, protein 32.9

Zucchini and Carrot Cakes

Prep time: 10 minutes I **Cooking time:** 10 minutes I **Servings:** 4

Ingredients:

- 1 yellow onion, chopped

- 2 zucchinis, grated

- 2 tablespoons almond flour

- 1 egg, whisked

- 1 garlic clove, minced

- A pinch of black pepper

- 1/3 cup carrot, shredded

- 1/3 cup cheddar, grated

- 1 tablespoon cilantro, chopped

- 1 teaspoon lemon zest, grated

- 2 tablespoons olive oil

Directions:

1. In a bowl, combine the zucchinis with the garlic, onion and the other ingredients except the oil, stir well and shape medium cakes out of this mix.

2. Heat up a pan with the oil over medium-high heat, add the zucchini cakes, cook for 5 minutes on each side, divide between plates and serve with a side salad.

Nutrition facts per serving: calories 271, fat 8.7, fiber 4, carbs 14.3, protein 4.6

Chickpeas Stew

Prep time: 10 minutes I **Cooking time:** 20 minutes I **Servings:** 4

Ingredients:

- 1 tablespoon olive oil

- 1 yellow onion, chopped

- 2 teaspoons chili powder

- 14 ounces chickpeas, cooked

- 14 ounces tomatoes, cubed

- 1 cup chicken stock

- 1 tablespoon cilantro, chopped

- A pinch of black pepper

Directions:

1. Heat up a pot with the oil over medium-high heat, add the onion and chili powder, stir and cook for 5 minutes.

2. Add the chickpeas and the other ingredients, toss, cook for 15 minutes over medium heat, divide into bowls and serve for lunch.

Nutrition facts per serving: calories 299, fat 13.2, fiber 4.7, carbs 17.2, protein 8.1

Chicken Salad

Prep time: 10 minutes I **Cooking time:** 0 minutes I **Servings:** 4

Ingredients:

- 1 tablespoon olive oil
- A pinch of black pepper
- 2 rotisserie chicken, skinless, boneless, shredded
- 1 pound cherry tomatoes, halved
- 1 red onion, chopped
- 4 cups baby spinach
- ¼ cup walnuts, chopped
- ½ teaspoon lemon zest, grated
- 2 tablespoons lemon juice

Directions:

1. In a salad bowl, combine the chicken with the tomato and the other ingredients, toss and serve for lunch.

Nutrition facts per serving: calories 349, fat 8.3, fiber 5.6, carbs 16.9, protein 22.8

Warm Asparagus Salad

Prep time: 10 minutes I **Cooking time:** 20 minutes I **Servings:** 4

Ingredients:

- 3 garlic cloves, minced

- 2 tablespoons olive oil

- 1 red onion, chopped

- 3 carrots, sliced

- ½ cup chicken stock

- 2 cups baby spinach

- 1 pound asparagus, trimmed and halved

- 1 red bell pepper, cut into strips

- 1 yellow bell pepper, cut into strips

- 1 green bell pepper, cut into strips

- A pinch of black pepper

Directions:

1. Heat up a pan with the oil over medium-high heat, add the onion and the garlic, stir and sauté for 2 minutes.

2. Add the asparagus and the other ingredients except the spinach, toss, and cook for 15 minutes.

3. Add the spinach, cook everything for 3 minutes more, divide into bowls and serve for lunch.

Nutrition facts per serving: calories 221, fat 11.2, fiber 3.4, carbs 14.3, protein 5.9

Beef Stew

Prep time: 10 minutes I **Cooking time:** 1 hour and 20 minutes I
Servings: 4

Ingredients:

- 1 pound beef stew meat, cubed

- 1 cup tomato sauce

- 1 cup beef stock

- 1 tablespoon olive oil

- 1 yellow onion, chopped

- ¼ teaspoon hot sauce

- 1 teaspoon onion powder

- 1 teaspoon garlic powder

- 1 tablespoon cilantro, chopped

Directions:

1. Heat up a pot with the oil over medium-high heat, add the meat and the onion, stir and brown for 5 minutes.

2. Add the tomato sauce and the rest of the ingredients, bring to a simmer and cook over medium heat for 1 hour and 15 minutes.

3. Divide into bowls and serve for lunch.

Nutrition facts per serving: calories 487, fat 15.3, fiber 5.8, carbs 56.3, protein 15

Rosemary Pork Chops

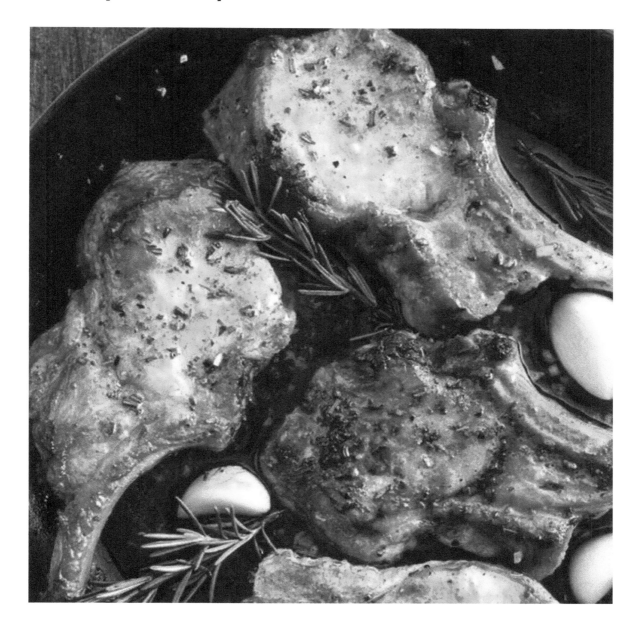

Prep time: 5 minutes I **Cooking time:** 8 hours and 10 minutes I
Servings: 4

Ingredients:

- 4 pork chops

- 1 tablespoon olive oil

- 2 shallots, chopped

- 1 pound white mushrooms, sliced

- ½ cup beef stock

- 1 tablespoon rosemary, chopped

- ¼ teaspoon garlic powder

- 1 teaspoon sweet paprika

Directions:

1. Heat up a pan with the oil over medium-high heat, add the pork chops and the shallots, toss, brown for 10 minutes and transfer to a slow cooker.

2. Add the rest of the ingredients, put the lid on and cook on Low for 8 hours.

3. Divide the pork chops and mushrooms between plates and serve for lunch.

Nutrition facts per serving: calories 349, fat 24, fiber 5.6, carbs 46.3, protein 17.5

Shrimp, Arugula and Coriander Salad

Prep time: 10 minutes I **Cooking time:** 8 minutes I **Servings:** 4

Ingredients:

- 1 tablespoon olive oil

- 1 red onion, sliced

- 1 pound shrimp, peeled and deveined

- 2 cups baby arugula

- 1 tablespoon balsamic vinegar

- 1 tablespoon lemon juice

- 1 tablespoon coriander, chopped

- A pinch of black pepper

Directions:

1. Heat up a pan with the oil over medium heat, add the onion, stir and sauté for 2 minutes.

2. Add the shrimp and the other ingredients, toss, cook for 6 minutes, divide into bowls and serve for lunch.

Nutrition facts per serving: calories 341, fat 11.5, fiber 3.8, carbs 17.3, protein 14.3

Eggplant and Tomato Stew

Prep time: 5 minutes I **Cooking time:** 20 minutes I **Servings:** 4

Ingredients:

- 1 pound eggplants, roughly cubed

- 2 garlic cloves, minced

- 2 tablespoons olive oil

- 1 yellow onion, chopped

- 1 teaspoon sweet paprika

- ½ cup cilantro, chopped

- 14 ounces tomatoes, chopped

- 1 tablespoon cilantro, chopped

Directions:

1. Heat up a pan with the oil over medium-high heat, add the onion and the garlic and sauté for 2 minutes.

2. Add the eggplant and the other ingredients except the cilantro, bring to a simmer and cook for 18 minutes.

3. Divide into bowls and serve with the cilantro sprinkled on top.

Nutrition facts per serving: calories 343, fat 12.3, fiber 3.7, carbs 16.56, protein 7.2

Parsley Beef and Peas Stew

Prep time: 10 minutes I **Cooking time:** 30 minutes I **Servings:** 4

Ingredients:

- 1 and ¼ cups beef stock

- 1 yellow onion, chopped

- 1 tablespoon olive oil

- 2 cups peas

- 1 pound beef stew meat, cubed

- 1 cup tomatoes, chopped

- 1 cup scallions, chopped

- ¼ cup parsley, chopped

- Black pepper to the taste

Directions:

1. Heat up a pot with the oil over medium-high heat, add the onion and the meat and brown for 5 minutes.

2. Add the peas and the other ingredients, stir, bring to a simmer and cook over medium heat for 25 minutes more.

3. Divide the mix into bowls and serve for lunch.

Nutrition facts per serving: calories 487, fat 15.4, fiber 4.6, carbs 44.6, protein 17.8

Lime Turkey Stew

Prep time: 5 minutes I **Cooking time:** 30 minutes I **Servings:** 4

Ingredients:

- 2 tablespoons olive oil

- 1 turkey breast, skinless, boneless and cubed

- 1 cup beef stock

- 1 cup tomato puree

- ¼ teaspoon lime zest, grated

- 1 yellow onion, chopped

- 1 tablespoon sweet paprika

- 1 tablespoon cilantro, chopped

- 2 tablespoons lime juice

- ¼ teaspoon ginger, grated

Directions:

1. Heat up a pot with the oil over medium-high heat, add the onion and the meat and brown for 5 minutes.

2. Add the stock and the other ingredients, bring to a simmer and cook over medium heat for 25 minutes.

3. Divide the mix into bowls and serve for lunch.

Nutrition facts per serving: calories 150, fat 8.1, fiber 2.7, carbs 12, protein 9.5

Beef and Black Beans Salad

Prep time: 10 minutes I **Cooking time:** 30 minutes I **Servings:** 4

Ingredients:

- 1 pound beef stew meat, cut into strips

- 1 tablespoon sage, chopped

- 1 tablespoon olive oil

- A pinch of black pepper

- ½ teaspoon cumin, ground

- 2 cups cherry tomatoes, cubed

- 1 avocado, peeled, pitted and cubed

- 1 cup black beans, cooked and drained

- ½ cup green onions, chopped

- 2 tablespoons lime juice

- 2 tablespoons balsamic vinegar

- 2 tablespoons cilantro, chopped

Directions:

1. Heat up a pan with the oil over medium-high heat, add the meat and brown for 5 minutes.

2. Add the sage, black pepper and the cumin, toss and cook for 5 minutes more.

3. Add the rest of the ingredients, toss, reduce heat to medium and cook the mix for 20 minutes.

4. Divide the salad into bowls and serve for lunch.

Nutrition facts per serving: calories 536, fat 21.4, fiber 12.5, carbs 40.4, protein 47

Squash and Peppers Mix

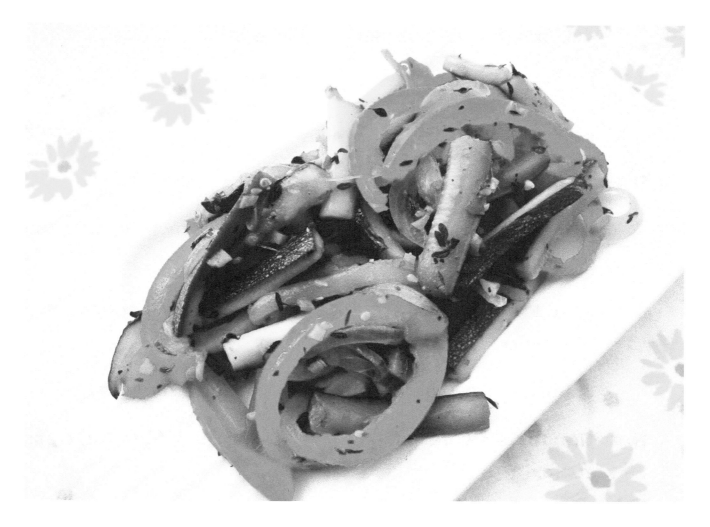

Prep time: 10 minutes I **Cooking time:** 20 minutes I **Servings:** 4

Ingredients:

- 1 pound squash, peeled and roughly cubed

- 1 cup chicken stock

- 1 cup tomatoes, crushed

- 1 tablespoon olive oil

- 1 red onion, chopped

- 2 orange sweet peppers, chopped

- ½ cup quinoa

- ½ tablespoon chives, chopped

Directions:

1. Heat up a pot with the oil over medium heat, add the onion, stir and sauté for 2 minutes.

2. Add the squash and the other ingredients, bring to a simmer, and cook for 15 minutes.

3. Stir the stew, divide into bowls and serve for lunch.

Nutrition facts per serving: calories 166, fat 5.3, fiber 4.7, carbs 26.3, protein 5.9

Beef, Green Onions and Peppers Mix

Prep time: 10 minutes I **Cooking time:** 20 minutes I **Servings:** 4

Ingredients:

- 1 green cabbage head, shredded

- ¼ cup beef stock

- 2 tomatoes, cubed

- 2 yellow onions, chopped

- ¾ cup red bell peppers, chopped

- 1 tablespoon olive oil

- 1 pound beef, ground

- ¼ cup cilantro, chopped

- ¼ cup green onions, chopped

- ¼ teaspoon red pepper, crushed

Directions:

1. Heat up a pan with the oil over medium heat, add the meat and the onions, stir and brown for 5 minutes.

2. Add the cabbage and the other ingredients, toss, cook for 15 minutes, divide into bowls and serve for lunch.

Nutrition facts per serving: calories 328, fat 11, fiber 6.9, carbs 20.1, protein 38.3

Pork, Green Beans and Tomato Stew

Prep time: 5 minutes I **Cooking time:** 8 hours and 10 minutes I
Servings: 4

Ingredients:

- 1 pound pork stew meat, cubed

- 1 tablespoon olive oil

- ½ pound green beans, trimmed and halved

- 2 yellow onions, chopped

- 2 garlic cloves, minced

- 2 cups beef stock

- 8 ounces tomato sauce

- A pinch of black pepper

- A pinch of allspice, ground

- 1 tablespoon rosemary, chopped

Directions:

1. Heat up a pan with the oil over medium-high heat, add the meat, garlic and onion, stir and brown for 10 minutes.

2. Transfer this to a slow cooker, add the other ingredients as well, put the lid on and cook on Low for 8 hours.

3. Divide the stew into bowls and serve.

Nutrition facts per serving: calories 334, fat 14.8, fiber 4.4, carbs 13.3, protein 36.7

Dill Zucchini Cream

Prep time: 10 minutes I **Cooking time:** 20 minutes I **Servings:** 4

Ingredients:

- 1 tablespoon olive oil

- 1 yellow onion, chopped

- 1 teaspoon ginger, grated

- 1 pound zucchinis, chopped

- 32 ounces chicken stock

- 1 cup coconut cream

- 1 tablespoon dill, chopped

Directions:

1. Heat up a pot with the oil over medium heat, add the onion and ginger, stir and cook for 5 minutes.

2. Add the zucchinis and the other ingredients, bring to a simmer and cook over medium heat for 15 minutes.

3. Blend using an immersion blender, divide into bowls and serve.

Nutrition facts per serving: calories 293, fat 12.3, fiber 2.7, carbs 11.2, protein 6.4

Shrimp, Walnuts and Grapes Bowls

Prep time: 5 minutes I **Cooking time:** 0 minutes I **Servings:** 4

Ingredients:

- 2 tablespoons mayonnaise

- 2 teaspoons chili powder

- A pinch of black pepper

- 1 pound shrimp, cooked, peeled and deveined

- 1 cup red grapes, halved

- ½ cup scallions, chopped

- ¼ cup walnuts, chopped

- 1 tablespoon cilantro, chopped

Directions:

1. In a salad bowl, combine shrimp with the chili powder and the other ingredients, toss and serve fro lunch.

Nutrition facts per serving: calories 298, fat 12.3, fiber 2.6, carbs 16.2, protein 7.8

Carrot and Celery Cream

Prep time: 5 minutes I **Cooking time:** 25 minutes I **Servings:** 4

Ingredients:

- 2 tablespoons olive oil

- 1 yellow onion, chopped

- 1 pound carrots, peeled and chopped

- 1 teaspoon turmeric powder

- 4 celery stalks, chopped

- 5 cups chicken stock

- A pinch of black pepper

- 1 tablespoon cilantro, chopped

Directions:

1. Heat up a pot with the oil over medium heat, add the onion, stir and sauté for 2 minutes.

2. Add the carrots and the other ingredients, bring to a simmer and cook over medium heat for 20 minutes.

3. Blend the soup using an immersion blender, ladle into bowls and serve.

Nutrition facts per serving: calories 221, fat 9.6, fiber 4.7, carbs 16, protein 4.8

Beef Soup

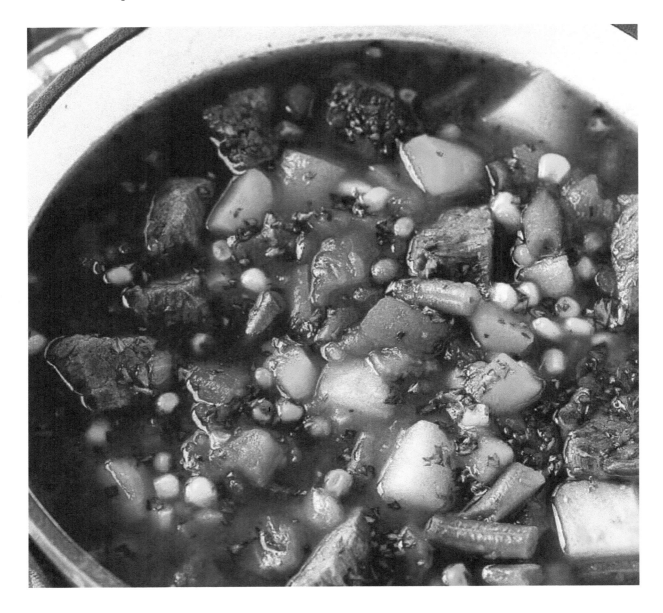

Prep time: 10 minutes I **Cooking time:** 1 hour and 40 minutes I
Servings: 4

Ingredients:

- 1 cup black beans, cooked

- 7 cups beef stock

- 1 green bell pepper, chopped

- 1 tablespoon olive oil

- 1 pound beef stew meat, cubed

- 1 yellow onion, chopped

- 3 garlic cloves, minced

- 1 chili pepper, chopped

- 1 potato, cubed

- A pinch of black pepper

- 1 tablespoon cilantro, chopped

Directions:

1. Heat up a pot with the oil over medium heat, add the onion, garlic and the meat, and brown for 5 minutes.

2. Add the beans and the rest of the ingredients except the cilantro, bring to a simmer and cook over medium heat for 1 hour and 35 minutes.

3. Add the cilantro, ladle the soup into bowls and serve.

Nutrition facts per serving: calories 421, fat 17.3, fiber 3.8, carbs 18.8, protein 23.5

Salmon and Salsa Bowls

Prep time: 10 minutes I **Cooking time:** 13 minutes I **Servings:** 4

Ingredients:

- ½ pound smoked salmon, boneless, skinless and cubed

- ½ pound shrimp, peeled and deveined

- 1 tablespoon olive oil

- 1 red onion, chopped

- ¼ cup tomatoes, cubed

- ½ cup mild salsa

- 2 tablespoons cilantro, chopped

Directions:

1. Heat up a pan with the oil over medium-high heat, add the salmon, toss and cook for 5 minutes.

2. Add the onion, shrimp and the other ingredients, cook for 7 minutes more, divide into bowls and serve.

Nutrition facts per serving: calories 251, fat 11.4, fiber 3.7, carbs 12.3, protein 7.1

Chicken and Herbs Sauce

Prep time: 5 minutes I **Cooking time:** 20 minutes I **Servings:** 4

Ingredients:

- 1 tablespoon olive oil

- 1 yellow onion, chopped

- A pinch of black pepper

- 1 pound chicken breasts, skinless, boneless and cubed

- 4 garlic cloves, minced

- 1 cup chicken stock

- 2 cups coconut cream

- 1 tablespoon basil, chopped

- 1 tablespoon chives, chopped

Directions:

1. Heat up a pan with the oil over medium-high heat, add the garlic, onion and the meat, toss and brown for 5 minutes.

2. Add the stock and the rest of the ingredients, bring to a simmer and cook over medium heat for 15 minutes.

3. Divide the mix between plates and serve.

Nutrition facts per serving: calories 451, fat 16.6, fiber 9, carbs 34.4, protein 34.5

Ginger Chicken and Veggies Stew

Prep time: 5 minutes I **Cooking time:** 20 minutes I **Servings:** 4

Ingredients:

- 1 pound chicken breasts, skinless, boneless and cubed

- 2 shallots, chopped

- 1 tablespoon olive oil

- 1 eggplant, cubed

- 1 cup tomatoes, crushed

- 1 tablespoon lime juice

- A pinch of black pepper

- ¼ teaspoon ginger, ground

- 1 tablespoon cilantro, chopped

Directions:

1. Heat up a pot with the oil over medium heat, add the shallots and the chicken and brown for 5 minutes.

2. Add the rest of the ingredients, bring to a simmer and cook over medium heat for 15 minutes more.

3. Divide into bowls and serve for lunch.

Nutrition facts per serving: calories 441, fat 14.6, fiber 4.9, carbs 44.4, protein 16.9

Chives Chicken and Endives

Prep time: 5 minutes I **Cooking time:** 20 minutes I **Servings:** 4

Ingredients:

- 1 pound chicken thighs, boneless, skinless and cubed

- 2 endives, shredded

- 1 cup chicken stock

- 1 tablespoon olive oil

- 1 yellow onion, chopped

- 1 carrot, sliced

- 2 garlic cloves, minced

- 8 ounces tomatoes, chopped

- 1 tablespoon chives, chopped

Directions:

1. Heat up a pan with the oil over medium-high heat, add the onion and garlic and sauté for 5 minutes.

2. Add the chicken and brown for 5 minutes more.

3. Add the rest of the ingredients, bring to a simmer, cook for 10 minutes more, divide between plates and serve.

Nutrition facts per serving: calories 411, fat 16.7, fiber 5.9, carbs 54.5, protein 24

Conclusion

Thank you for making it throughout, it would behave to have feedback of your feelings relating to these fast dishes to remain in form without having to quit the satisfaction of eating your preferred recipes.

Keep in mind that this diet regimen does not just aim at slimming but likewise at physical wellness, try to find the best method to trigger your metabolism, as well as remember that this diet regimen is a genuine anti-aging program, the charm of these snak and dessert recipes will certainly permit you to have fun and also drop weight at the same time as well as this will allow you to lose weight in a calm as well as loosened up way without having to reduce on your own to a circumstance of stress and also irritation.

Enjoy and also appreciate your diet plan.

CPSIA information can be obtained
at www.ICGtesting.com
Printed in the USA
LVHW062100020621
689026LV00019B/1460